KEEP YOUR BONES STRONG

Practical Approach to Osteoporosis, Improve Bone Strength and Reduce Your Risk of Fractures

DR. EDWARD M. TAYLOR

KEEP YOUR BONES STRONG

Practical Approach to Osteoporosis, Improve Bone Strength and Reduce Your Risk of Fractures

Dr. Edward M. Taylor

Table Of Contents

Introduction

Welcome to "Keep Your Bones Strong: Practical Approach to Osteoporosis, Improve Bone Strength and Reduce Your Risk of Fractures" – a comprehensive guide tailored just for you, the reader who seeks not just information, but understanding; not just guidance, but a roadmap to better bone health and a vibrant life. In the pages that follow, you will embark on a journey of discovery, empowerment, and transformation, as we delve into the intricate world of osteoporosis – a condition that affects millions of lives but is often misunderstood.

In the fast-paced rhythm of modern life, health often takes a back seat. But your bones, those silent sentinels beneath your skin, deserve your attention. Imagine this: a life where every movement is not just painless but a source of strength. Imagine standing tall, knowing that your bones are robust, resilient, and reliable. This book is your ticket to turning that imagination into reality. Whether you're young or old, male or female, osteoporosis does not discriminate, and neither does this book. It's for everyone who wants to understand the whispers of their bones, decode the language of their body, and respond with informed decisions.

Why should you care about osteoporosis? Because your bones are the foundation upon which your entire life is built. They support you, quite literally, every step of the way. They are the scaffolding that allows you to explore the world, embrace your loved ones, and relish the experiences that make life meaningful. Osteoporosis, often called the silent thief, can erode this foundation quietly, leading to fractures, pain, and a loss of independence. But fear not, for this book is your shield against this thief. Here, you will find not only the reasons behind osteoporosis but also the strategies to fortify your bones and diminish the risk of fractures.

How often have you wished for a healthier, more active life? How frequently have you yearned to understand your body better, to nurture it in a way that fosters longevity and vitality? Your desire for a life less burdened by the fear of fragile bones is the driving force behind this book. Here, you will discover the desire for strength met with the tools to achieve it. From dietary secrets that promote bone density to exercises that enhance your posture and balance, this book offers a treasure trove of knowledge. The desire for independence is met with chapters dedicated to adapting your lifestyle and surroundings, ensuring that your home is a sanctuary of safety and support.

The time for action is now. With every page you turn, you'll gain insights that empower you to take charge of your bone health. No longer will osteoporosis be a daunting specter; instead, it will be a challenge you can face head-on, armed with knowledge and determination. As you read on, you will find practical tips, actionable advice, and real-life stories that inspire you to make positive changes. From understanding diagnostic tests to exploring medical treatments and embracing lifestyle modifications, this book equips you with the tools to transform your desires into actions.

So, let the journey begin. Open your mind and heart to the wealth of information within these pages. Let this book be your companion, guiding you toward a future where your bones are not just strong, but unbreakable; where your life is not just lived, but celebrated in all its vibrant glory. Together, let's embark on this transformative odyssey toward better bone health, greater strength, and a life filled with vitality.

Chapter 1: Understanding Osteoporosis

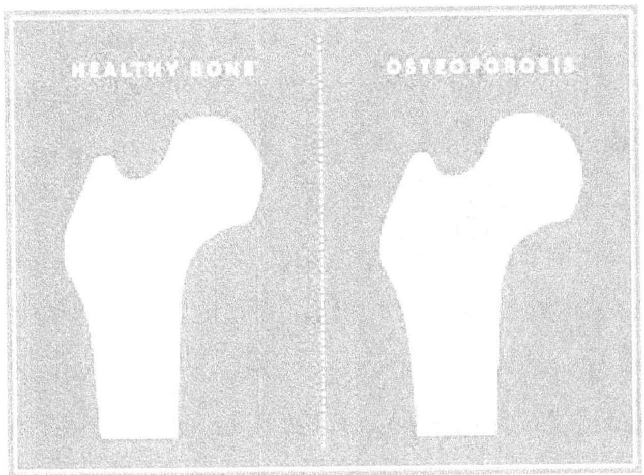

Osteoporosis, a term derived from the Greek words "osteo" meaning bone and "porosis" meaning porous, is a silent and often underestimated health concern affecting millions worldwide. In this comprehensive exploration, we will unravel the complexities of osteoporosis, delving into its definition, causes, and the crucial factors that underscore the importance of bone health in our lives.

Definition and Causes

To truly comprehend osteoporosis, one must first grasp its essence. Osteoporosis is a bone disorder characterized by decreased bone mass and structural deterioration of bone tissue, leading to fragile bones and an increased susceptibility to fractures. In simpler terms, it weakens the bones, making them more prone to breakage, even from minor falls or accidents. This condition, often referred to as a "silent disease," develops gradually over years, with no noticeable symptoms until a fracture occurs.

The causes of osteoporosis are multifaceted, encompassing a blend of genetic, lifestyle, and hormonal factors. One primary cause is an imbalance in the bone remodeling process, where the body absorbs old bone tissue faster than it can replace it with new, sturdy bone. This imbalance can be attributed to aging, hormonal changes, and nutritional deficiencies.

Postmenopausal women and elderly individuals are particularly susceptible due to decreased estrogen levels, which play a pivotal role in maintaining bone density. Additionally, a sedentary lifestyle, lack of physical activity, smoking, excessive alcohol consumption, and certain medical conditions or medications can exacerbate the risk of osteoporosis.

Optional reasons for osteoporosis in grown-ups

The accompanying drugs, conditions and surgeries can speed up bone misfortune, expanding your gamble of osteoporosis. Check with your PCP about different meds or conditions that might influence your bone misfortune too.

Prescriptions
- Steroids
- Anticonvulsants

- Extreme thyroid prescription
- Certain diuretics, like circle diuretics
- Certain blood thinners, like heparin and warfarin
- Certain compound inhibitors, for example, aromatase inhibitors
- Prescriptions used to treat bosom and prostate malignant growths

Ailments

Endocrine issues
- Sex chemical lack (hypogonadism)
- Extreme parathyroid chemical (hyperparathyroidism)
- Cushing condition
- Type 1 and type 2 diabetes

Stomach, digestive and liver problems
- Crohn's sickness
- Celiac sickness
- Essential biliary cirrhosis

- Lactose prejudice

- Rheumatoid joint pain
- Inability to bleed (amenorrhea)
- Loss of motion or drawn out bed rest because of an ailment

Surgeries

- Organ relocate
- Gastric and upper digestive medical procedures

Risk Factors

Understanding the risk factors associated with osteoporosis is paramount in its prevention and early detection. While aging is an inevitable risk factor, there are several other variables that influence an individual's vulnerability to this condition.

1. **Genetics:** A family history of osteoporosis significantly elevates the risk. If your parents or

siblings have suffered from this condition, it is crucial to be proactive in bone health management.

2. Gender: Women, especially after menopause, are at higher risk due to the rapid decline in estrogen levels. However, men are not exempt; they can also develop osteoporosis, although typically at a later age.

3. Nutritional Deficiencies: Inadequate intake of calcium, vitamin D, and other essential nutrients weakens bones. Calcium is the building block of bones, and vitamin D aids in its absorption. A deficiency in either can compromise bone health.

4. Physical Inactivity: Bones, like muscles, require regular exercise to stay strong. Lack of weight-bearing activities, such as walking, dancing, or weightlifting, diminishes bone density.

5. Hormonal Imbalances: Conditions like hyperthyroidism or hormonal treatments for various ailments can disrupt the delicate balance of hormones responsible for bone maintenance.

6. Medications: Long-term use of certain medications, such as corticosteroids and some anticonvulsants, can negatively impact bone density.

7. Body Composition: Individuals with low body weight or a petite frame have less bone mass to lose before reaching a critical point, making them more vulnerable to fractures.

Signs And Symptoms

Osteoporosis is frequently alluded to as a quiet illness since bone misfortune happens easily over numerous years. And, surprisingly, in cases when the misfortune is unusually quick, during the beginning phases you may not encounter any signs or side effects.

Then, at that point, at some point, you break a bone while doing a standard errand — perhaps you break a rib while lifting the clothing bin or crack a vertebra while bowing down to tie your shoes. As of now, the illness may currently be deeply grounded and portions of your skeleton may as of now be very feeble and vulnerable to break.

Different signs and side effects might happen on the off chance that you've encountered a pressure

Crack of the spine, including:
- Back torment
- Deficiency of level
- Stooped act

Recollect that back aggravation, deficiency of level or stooped act doesn't mean you have osteoporosis. Provided that you've encountered a pressure crack does the illness by and large produce back torment. The most well-known reasons for back torment are muscle strain and circle injury. In any case, since there's the likelihood that back aggravation could originate from an osteoporosis-related crack, it means a lot to see a specialist to decide the reason and make a fitting move.

In the beginning phases of osteoporosis, there may be no signs that you have the sickness. Along these lines, it's vital to know about factors that put you at expanded risk. Assuming you're worried that you might have an increased chance of the illness, talk with your PCP about whether you ought to have a bone thickness test. Keep in mind, the best opportunity to act is before you break a bone —not later.

TYPES

Osteoporosis occurs for various reasons. To pick the right course of treatment, your PCP will need to decide the sort of osteoporosis you have and what caused it.

In ladies, osteoporosis most frequently results from bone misfortune that happens after menopause. Frequently, it's a blend of postmenopausal bone misfortune and age-related bone misfortune that causes the condition. Most grown-ups arrive at their pinnacle bone mass in their late 20s or mid 30s. They continuously lose bone mass in the years that follow.

Bone misfortune might happen because of another infection or from the utilization of specific meds. This kind of bone misfortune can prompt optional types of osteoporosis — because of causes beyond the ordinary impacts of maturing. Be that as it may, auxiliary osteoporosis is more uncommon.

Postmenopausal osteoporosis

Postmenopausal osteoporosis occurs soon after menopause as levels of the chemical estrogen decline. In most ladies, menopause happens around age 50. A few years before a lady encounters her last monthly cycle, estrogen levels are as of now beginning to drop. The decrease go on for one more three to four years after the last cycle. During this time, bone misfortune speeds up on the grounds that estrogen, which is expected to keep up with bone wellbeing, is as of now not present at adequate levels. Ladies can lose up to 10% or a greater amount of their bone mass during the five to seven years after menopause.

In ladies around age 70, bone misfortune eases back however doesn't stop. By their 80s, ladies might have lost 35% to half of their bone mass. Assuming that you enter menopause with low bone mass, or on the other hand assuming that you quickly lose bone after menopause, you're bound to foster osteoporosis. That is the reason it's vital to do whatever it may take to fabricate bone mass in your initial years and keep up with it as a grown-up.

Men get osteoporosis, as well

While ladies might be most in danger, men likewise get osteoporosis. Starting in their mid-30s men might begin to lose bone mass at a pace of up to around 1% every year. By around age 70 they lose bone mass at a comparable rate as ladies do.

Numerous men might consider osteoporosis an infection that influences ladies and overlook basic moves toward assist with forestalling it. Truth be told, around 2 million men in the US have osteoporosis, and another 12 million are in danger of getting it. It's assessed that up to 25% of men more established than age 50 will break a bone because of osteoporosis. In the U.S. Around 80,000 hip cracks every year happen in men.

Age-related osteoporosis

All people — ladies and men — lose bone with age. Losing a little level of bone mass every year up to maturity 80 is typical. This happens on the grounds that as you age, new bone arrangement eases back while bone breakdown remains something similar or increments. The inner construction of your bones likewise debilitates, and the external shell diminishes. These improvements are each of the a typical piece of maturing, which occurs at an alternate rate for everybody. What's significant is the level of progress.

Osteoporosis is most normal in more seasoned ladies in light of the fact that their skeletons experience a one-two punch. Notwithstanding age-related bone misfortune, which influences all kinds of people, numerous more seasoned ladies have previously experienced bone misfortune from menopause.

Optional reasons for osteoporosis

At times osteoporosis might be connected with specific circumstances, techniques or drugs that speed up bone misfortune. Optional causes are a component in around 20% to 30% of postmenopausal ladies with osteoporosis and around half of ladies who are moving toward menopause (perimenopausal). Among men with osteoporosis, around half have an optional reason. Osteoporosis that is reasonable because of one of these causes is known as auxiliary osteoporosis.

As a rule, the more youthful you are the point at which you get a finding of osteoporosis, the more probable it is that an optional element is adding to the issue. The sidebar above records a portion of the more normal variables related with optional osteoporosis.

Importance of Bone Health

Bones, often taken for granted, are the sturdy pillars that support our body and enable movement. Beyond their structural role, bones serve as a reservoir for essential minerals, including calcium and phosphorus, which are vital for various physiological functions. Understanding the profound significance of bone health is crucial for overall well-being.

1. Structural Support: Bones provide the framework that allows us to stand, walk, run, and perform everyday activities. A robust skeletal system ensures stability and balance, reducing the risk of falls and fractures.

2. Protection of Organs: Bones, especially the skull and ribcage, safeguard vital organs like the brain, heart, and lungs from external trauma, ensuring their proper functioning.

3. Mineral Storage: Bones store minerals, such as calcium and phosphorus, which are released into the bloodstream as needed to maintain the body's mineral balance. Calcium, in particular, is essential for muscle function, blood clotting, and nerve transmission.

4. Blood Cell Formation: Within the bone marrow, specialized cells produce red blood cells, white blood cells, and platelets. These cells are indispensable for oxygen transport, immune defense, and clotting, respectively.

5. Endocrine Regulation: Bones secrete osteocalcin, a hormone that influences insulin sensitivity and energy expenditure. This underlines the intricate connection between bone health and metabolic processes.

6. Longevity and Quality of Life: Healthy bones contribute significantly to longevity and a higher quality of life. By preserving bone density and strength, individuals can maintain their independence and mobility well into their senior years.

In this in-depth exploration of osteoporosis, we've journeyed through the intricacies of its definition, causes, and the fundamental importance of bone health. Armed with this knowledge, you are better equipped to make informed decisions that can safeguard your bones and enhance your overall well-being.

Remember, your bones are remarkable structures, resilient yet fragile, and deserving of your attention and care. By embracing a balanced diet rich in calcium and vitamin D, engaging in regular physical activity, avoiding harmful habits like smoking and excessive alcohol consumption, and being mindful of your overall health, you can fortify your bones and reduce the risk of osteoporosis.

As you embark on your path to optimal bone health, let this newfound understanding be your guiding light. Cherish your bones, nurture them, and they will support you in a life filled with vitality, strength, and endless possibilities. Here's to strong bones, and here's to a future where you can live your life to the fullest, unburdened by the fear of fragility.

Chapter 2: Bone Basics

Welcome to Chapter 2 of "Keep Your Bones Strong: Practical Approach to Osteoporosis, Improve Bone Strength and Reduce Your Risk of Fractures." In this chapter, we embark on a fascinating journey into the intricate world of bone biology. Understanding the fundamentals of your skeletal system is the first step toward building a strong foundation for a healthier life. So, let's dive deep into the nuances of bones, exploring their structure, function, density, and mass, unraveling the mysteries that lie beneath your skin.

2.1 The Skeletal System

The human body is a marvel of engineering, and at its core lies the skeletal system – the framework that supports and protects your body's organs, muscles, and tissues. Imagine it as a complex network of interconnected structures, akin to the framework of a well-built house. Your bones are not just lifeless structures; they are dynamic, living tissues that undergo constant remodeling and repair.

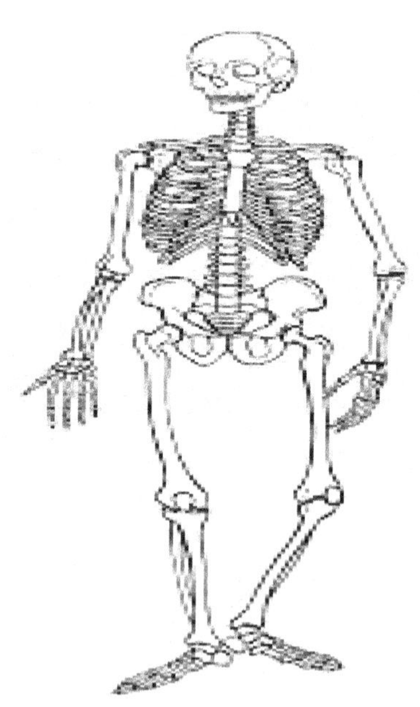

Structure and Function of Bones

Bones come in various shapes and sizes, each designed for specific functions. Long bones, such as the femur and humerus, provide support and enable movement. Short bones, like those in your wrists and ankles, offer stability and support. Flat bones, including the skull and shoulder blades, protect vital organs like the brain and heart. Irregular bones, such as those in your spine, have unique shapes tailored to their specific roles.

The structure of bones is a marvel in itself. Picture a cross-section of bone, and you'll see a dense outer layer called cortical bone, providing strength and protection. Beneath this lies trabecular bone, a spongy network resembling a honeycomb. This spongy structure adds strength without unnecessary weight, making bones both lightweight and sturdy.

Beyond providing a framework, bones serve as reservoirs for essential minerals, primarily calcium and phosphorus. These minerals are not just static deposits; they are in constant flux, released into the bloodstream as needed for various bodily functions, including muscle contractions and nerve signaling. Additionally, bones house bone marrow, a vital component of your body's blood-forming system, responsible for producing red and white blood cells.

Bone Density and Bone Mass

Now, let's delve into the concepts of bone density and bone mass, which are pivotal in understanding osteoporosis. Bone density refers to the amount of mineral content in bone tissue. It is a measure of how compact and strong your bones are. Think of bone density as the 'quality' of your bones – denser bones are less prone to fractures and injuries.

Bone mass, on the other hand, refers to the total amount of bone tissue in your body. It is influenced by various factors, including genetics, diet, physical activity, and hormonal balance. Throughout your life, your body continuously builds new bone tissue to replace old or damaged bone in a process known as remodeling. During childhood and adolescence, bone formation outpaces breakdown, leading to an increase in bone mass. However, as you age, especially after the age of 30, the balance shifts, and bone breakdown may surpass formation, resulting in a decline in bone mass.

Understanding your bone density and mass is crucial because it directly correlates with your risk of developing osteoporosis. Individuals with lower bone density are at a higher risk of fractures, as their bones lack the necessary strength and resilience to withstand the stresses of daily activities.

In the next sections of this chapter, we will explore how bone density is measured, the factors that influence bone health, and strategies to enhance and maintain your bone density and mass throughout life. By the end of this chapter, you will have a profound understanding of the intricate world of bones, setting the stage for your journey toward stronger, healthier bones.

In this section, we delved into the fundamentals of the skeletal system, exploring the structure and function of bones, as well as the concepts of bone density and bone mass. Armed with this knowledge, you are better equipped to comprehend the subsequent chapters, where we will unravel the complexities of osteoporosis and empower you with the tools to safeguard your bone health.

So, stay tuned as we continue our exploration into the realm of osteoporosis, uncovering valuable insights that will pave the way for a future of strong and resilient bones.

2.2 How Bones Grow and Change

Bones, the sturdy framework of our bodies, are remarkable in their ability to adapt, grow, and change throughout our lives. Understanding the intricate processes of bone development, remodeling, and the effects of aging is crucial in appreciating the significance of maintaining optimal bone health.

Bone Development in Childhood and Adolescence

In the early stages of life, bones undergo a rapid and dynamic growth process. This period, primarily during childhood and adolescence, is pivotal for establishing strong and healthy bones that will support an individual throughout their lifetime.

During childhood, bones grow in both length and width. Long bones, such as those in the arms and legs, have growth plates located near their ends. These growth plates consist of cartilage cells that divide and eventually harden into bone tissue. This process, known as ossification, leads to an increase in bone length. Simultaneously, bones widen as new bone material is added to the outer surface.

Adolescence marks a significant growth spurt, with hormones playing a crucial role. Growth hormone stimulates the growth plates, triggering the rapid increase in height observed during this period. Additionally, sex hormones, such as estrogen and testosterone, contribute to bone growth and mineralization. Adequate nutrition, especially calcium and vitamin D, is essential during these years, as deficiencies can hinder proper bone development, potentially leading to weakened bones later in life.

Bone Remodeling in Adulthood

As we transition into adulthood, our bones do not remain static; they constantly undergo a process called bone remodeling. This remarkable mechanism ensures that bones remain strong and adaptive to the body's changing needs.

Bone remodeling involves two essential phases: resorption and formation. During resorption, specialized cells called osteoclasts break down old or damaged bone tissue. This process is essential for removing worn-out bone and making space for new, healthier bone to form. Osteoclasts release enzymes that dissolve the bone matrix, allowing minerals like calcium and phosphorus to be released back into the bloodstream.

Following resorption, the bone formation phase begins. Osteoblasts, another type of specialized bone cell, move in to create new bone tissue. They produce collagen, a protein that forms the framework for the new bone, and facilitate the mineralization process by depositing calcium and other minerals onto the collagen matrix. This dynamic balance between resorption and formation ensures the structural integrity of bones and their ability to adapt to mechanical stress.

Effects of Aging on Bones

As we age, the balance between bone resorption and formation becomes disrupted, leading to several changes in bone structure and density. One of the primary consequences of aging is a decrease in bone mass and density, a condition known as osteopenia. In more severe cases, this condition progresses to osteoporosis, characterized by significantly weakened bones that are susceptible to fractures even with minor trauma.

Several factors contribute to the effects of aging on bones:

1. Hormonal Changes: With aging, levels of estrogen and testosterone decline. These hormones play a significant role in maintaining bone density. In postmenopausal women, the drop in estrogen levels accelerates bone loss, making them more vulnerable to osteoporosis.

2. Reduced Calcium Absorption: As we age, our bodies become less efficient at absorbing calcium from the diet, leading to decreased mineralization of bone tissue.

3. **Physical Inactivity:** Lack of weight-bearing exercises and physical inactivity can accelerate bone loss. Bones need mechanical stress, such as that generated during walking or weightlifting, to maintain their density and strength.

4. Nutritional Deficiencies: Inadequate intake of calcium, vitamin D, and other essential nutrients can compromise bone health, especially in the elderly.

5. Chronic Health Conditions: Certain medical conditions, such as rheumatoid arthritis and hormonal disorders, can impact bone health. Additionally, long-term use of medications like corticosteroids can lead to bone loss.

6. Genetic Factors: Genetic predisposition plays a role in determining bone density and susceptibility to osteoporosis. Individuals with a family history of the condition are at a higher risk.

7. Changes in Bone Structure: With aging, bones may undergo structural changes, such as decreased trabecular bone (the spongy bone tissue inside bones) and increased porosity, making them more fragile and prone to fractures.

In understanding how bones grow, adapt, and change over a lifetime, we gain valuable insights into the importance of proactive bone health management. By recognizing the factors that influence bone development, remodeling, and the effects of aging, we can take informed steps to mitigate risks and maintain strong, resilient bones. As we delve deeper into this knowledge, the subsequent chapters of this book will equip you with practical strategies, lifestyle modifications, and medical insights to safeguard your bones and embark on a journey towards a life filled with vitality and mobility. Remember, your bones are the foundation upon which your active, fulfilling life stands – let's ensure that foundation remains unshakable.

Chapter 3: Diagnosing Osteoporosis

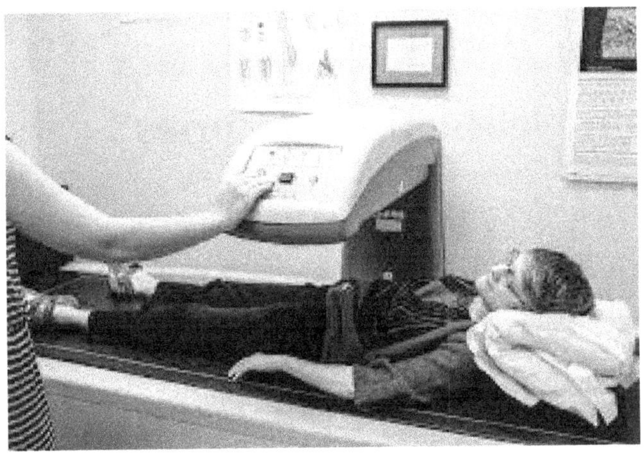

In the labyrinth of osteoporosis diagnosis, understanding the tools and techniques available is paramount. In this chapter, we will unravel the intricate web of diagnostics, focusing on the gold standard – Bone Density Tests. These tests not only decode the current state of your bone health but also provide crucial insights into your future well-being.

Prepare to journey deep into the realm of diagnostics, where knowledge is not just power but a shield against the silent progression of osteoporosis.

3.1 Bone Density Tests: Unraveling the Mysteries

Bone density tests, also known as bone mineral density (BMD) tests, are instrumental in diagnosing osteoporosis and assessing the risk of fractures. These tests measure the amount of minerals, primarily calcium, in a specific segment of bone. By doing so, they provide valuable information about bone strength and density, enabling healthcare professionals to make informed decisions regarding your bone health.

The Gold Standard: Dual-Energy X-ray Absorptiometry (DEXA) Scan

The Marvel of DEXA:

At the heart of osteoporosis diagnosis lies the marvel of medical technology – the Dual-Energy X-ray Absorptiometry (DEXA) scan. This non-invasive and painless procedure is the gold standard for measuring bone density. During a DEXA scan, low-level X-rays pass through the bones, detecting the amount of X-ray energy that is absorbed by the bone tissue. This information is then processed by a computer to generate precise and detailed images of your bones.

Understanding T-Score and Z-Score:

The results of a DEXA scan are typically presented in two essential metrics: T-score and Z-score. The T-score compares your bone density to that of a healthy young adult, providing a clear indication of your bone health status. A T-score of -1 and above is considered normal, while a score between -1 and -2.5 indicates osteopenia (low bone density). A T-score of -2.5 or lower signifies osteoporosis.

The Z-score, on the other hand, compares your bone density to that of individuals of your age, gender, and size. A Z-score significantly below the average for your demographic may indicate underlying health conditions or the need for further investigation.

Beyond DEXA: Exploring Other Diagnostic Methods

While DEXA scans are highly reliable, there are other diagnostic methods that healthcare professionals may employ to gather a comprehensive understanding of your bone health.

Quantitative Computed Tomography (QCT):

QCT is another imaging technique that provides detailed images of bones. It measures bone mineral content and density, offering valuable information about the structural integrity of your bones. QCT is particularly useful in assessing the spine and can detect subtle changes in bone density.

Peripheral Dual-Energy X-ray Absorptiometry (pDEXA) and Quantitative Ultrasound (QUS):

These portable and cost-effective devices are used to assess bone density in peripheral skeletal sites such as the heel or wrist. While they may not be as precise as central DEXA scans, they offer a quick and convenient way to estimate bone density, especially in locations where access to advanced diagnostic equipment is limited.

Magnetic Resonance Imaging (MRI) and Computed Tomography (CT) Scans:

In certain cases, healthcare professionals may recommend MRI or CT scans to evaluate bone health. These imaging techniques can provide detailed information about bone structure, helping diagnose osteoporosis-related fractures and assessing bone quality.

As you journey through the realm of osteoporosis diagnosis, remember that knowledge is your strongest ally. Understanding the nuances of bone density tests equips you with the power to advocate for your own health. Whether it's the precision of a DEXA scan or the accessibility of peripheral methods, each diagnostic tool serves a unique purpose, guiding healthcare professionals toward accurate diagnoses and personalized treatment plans.

Armed with this knowledge, you can approach osteoporosis diagnosis with confidence, knowing that you have a firm grasp on the methods used to assess your bone health. The path to stronger bones and a vibrant life begins with awareness, and in the world of osteoporosis, awareness starts with understanding the tools that shape your diagnosis. Embrace this knowledge, for it empowers you to make informed decisions, take proactive measures, and embark on a journey toward healthier, more resilient bones.

3.2 Interpreting Bone Density Results

When it comes to understanding your bone health, deciphering the results of bone density tests is crucial. In this section, we will unravel the complexities of bone density results, focusing on two essential components: the T-Score and the Z-Score. By the end of this comprehensive exploration, you will not only comprehend the meaning behind these scores but also gain valuable insights into your diagnosis, empowering you to make informed decisions about your bone health.

The T-Score: Decoding Your Bone Density

The T-Score is a fundamental aspect of bone density testing, providing a numerical value that compares your bone density to that of a healthy young adult of the same gender. A T-Score below -1.0 indicates a bone density that is lower than the young adult average, signifying a potential risk of osteoporosis. The lower the T-Score, the greater the risk.

Understanding T-Score Categories

1. Normal Range (T-Score above -1.0): If your T-Score falls within this range, your bone density is considered normal, indicating a lower risk of fractures. However, maintaining a healthy lifestyle and monitoring your bone health is still essential to prevent future issues.

2. Osteopenia (T-Score between -1.0 and -2.5): This category suggests low bone density, which is a precursor to osteoporosis. Individuals in this range have a higher risk of fractures. However, the condition is reversible with proper intervention, such as dietary changes, exercise, and sometimes medications.

3. Osteoporosis (T-Score below -2.5): A T-Score below -2.5 confirms an osteoporosis diagnosis, indicating significantly reduced bone density and an increased risk of fractures. Medical intervention, lifestyle modifications, and sometimes medication are necessary to manage this condition effectively.

Factors Affecting T-Score Accuracy

Several factors can influence your T-Score, such as age, gender, and race. It's crucial for your healthcare provider to consider these factors when interpreting your results, ensuring a more accurate assessment of your bone health. Additionally, certain medical conditions and medications can affect bone density, warranting a comprehensive evaluation of your overall health.

The Z-Score: Contextualizing Your Results

While the T-Score compares your bone density to that of a young adult, the Z-Score compares your bone density to that of individuals in your age group, providing a more contextually relevant assessment.

Understanding Z-Score Categories

1. Within Expected Range (Z-Score above -1.0): A Z-Score within this range indicates that your bone density is typical for your age group, suggesting no significant cause for concern. However, it's essential to maintain healthy lifestyle habits to support your bone health as you age.

2. Below Expected Range (Z-Score below -1.0): A Z-Score below -1.0 suggests that your bone density is lower than expected for your age, indicating potential underlying issues. Further investigation is necessary to identify the cause, which may include medical conditions or medications affecting bone health.

Understanding Your Diagnosis: Beyond the Numbers

While the T-Score and Z-Score provide valuable numerical data, understanding your diagnosis goes beyond these figures. Your healthcare provider will consider various factors, such as your medical history, lifestyle, and overall health, to create a comprehensive picture of your bone health.

Medical History Assessment

Your healthcare provider will inquire about your medical history, including past fractures, family history of osteoporosis, and any underlying medical conditions that might affect bone health. This information helps in understanding the potential causes of your bone density results.

Lifestyle Evaluation:

Your lifestyle habits, including diet, physical activity, smoking, and alcohol consumption, play a significant role in bone health. A balanced diet rich in calcium and vitamin D, coupled with regular weight-bearing exercises, can positively impact your bone density. Your healthcare provider will assess these factors to determine if lifestyle modifications are necessary.

Additional Diagnostic Tests

In some cases, additional tests may be required to investigate underlying causes of low bone density. Blood tests to assess vitamin and mineral levels, hormone levels, and thyroid function can provide valuable insights. Your healthcare provider might also recommend imaging tests, such as X-rays or MRI scans, to evaluate your bones further.

Consultation with Specialists:

Depending on the severity of your condition and underlying factors, your healthcare provider may refer you to specialists such as endocrinologists or rheumatologists. These specialists have expertise in bone health and can conduct in-depth assessments to tailor a suitable treatment plan for your specific needs.

Personalized Treatment and Prevention Plans

Once your diagnosis is thoroughly understood, your healthcare provider will collaborate with you to create a personalized treatment and prevention plan. This plan may include a combination of dietary changes, exercise routines, medications, and regular follow-ups to monitor your progress. It's essential to actively engage in this process, adhering to the recommended treatments and lifestyle modifications to improve your bone health effectively.

In conclusion, interpreting bone density results involves more than just understanding the T-Score and Z-Score. It encompasses a holistic evaluation of your medical history, lifestyle choices, and additional diagnostic tests, all aimed at providing a comprehensive understanding of your bone health. Armed with this knowledge, you are not merely a passive recipient of information but an active participant in your journey toward stronger, healthier bones.

Remember, your bone health is within your control. By understanding your diagnosis, embracing a proactive approach to your well-being, and collaborating closely with your healthcare provider, you can take significant strides toward preserving and enhancing your bone density. This understanding empowers you to make informed decisions, paving the way for a future where your bones remain resilient and your life remains vibrant.

As you move forward on this journey, carry with you the knowledge that you are equipped with the tools to nurture your bone health. Embrace the changes, celebrate the victories, and revel in the strength of your bones. Your commitment to understanding your diagnosis is the first step toward a life where fractures are minimized, and vitality knows no bounds. Embrace this knowledge, and let it guide you toward a future where your bones support you, allowing you to live life to the fullest.

Chapter 4: Prevention and Lifestyle Strategies

In the pursuit of strong and resilient bones, nutrition plays a pivotal role. This chapter explores the essential elements your body craves to fortify its skeletal structure, emphasizing not just the significance of calcium and vitamin D but also shedding light on other crucial nutrients that contribute to your overall bone health.

4.1 Nutrition for Strong Bones

Your body is a complex and finely tuned machine, and its performance depends significantly on the nutrients you provide. When it comes to bones, calcium and vitamin D take the spotlight as the dynamic duo essential for maintaining bone density and strength.

Importance of Calcium and Vitamin D

Calcium is the cornerstone of bone health. It's the mineral that lends bones their strength and rigidity, akin to the sturdy framework of a house. Without an adequate supply of calcium, bones can become brittle and prone to fractures. Imagine calcium as the builder, laying the foundation for healthy bones and teeth. While dairy products like milk, cheese, and yogurt are renowned for their calcium content, other sources include leafy green vegetables, fortified foods, and certain types of fish. Ensuring a balanced intake of calcium throughout life is pivotal, especially during childhood and adolescence when bones are growing rapidly, and in adulthood to maintain bone mass.

Vitamin D

Often dubbed the sunshine vitamin, vitamin D is unique because your body can produce it when exposed to sunlight. Vitamin D plays a vital role in calcium absorption, acting as a facilitator that ensures calcium finds its way into your bones where it's needed most. Without sufficient vitamin D, even if you consume ample calcium, your body might struggle to absorb it effectively. Besides sunlight, dietary sources of vitamin D include fatty fish, egg yolks, and fortified products like cereals and milk. For those living in regions with limited sunlight, vitamin D supplements might be necessary to meet the body's requirements.

Other Essential Nutrients

While calcium and vitamin D are the stars of the show, they don't work alone. Several other nutrients are integral to the bone health narrative:

Vitamin K:

Vitamin K aids in bone mineralization and supports the regulation of calcium within bones and blood vessels. Leafy greens, broccoli, and Brussels sprouts are rich sources of vitamin K, contributing to the overall matrix of bone health.

Magnesium:

Magnesium participates in bone structure by influencing the activities of osteoblasts and osteoclasts, the cells responsible for building and breaking down bone tissue. Nuts, seeds, whole grains, and green leafy vegetables are magnesium-packed options.

Phosphorus:

Phosphorus, alongside calcium, contributes to bone strength. It's abundant in protein-rich foods like meat, fish, dairy, and nuts. A balanced intake of phosphorus ensures that your bones have a robust support system.

Protein:

Proteins provide the amino acids necessary for building and repairing tissues, including bones. Incorporating lean meats, poultry, fish, beans, and legumes into your diet ensures a healthy supply of protein, aiding in bone maintenance and growth.

Trace Minerals:

Trace minerals such as zinc, copper, and manganese are involved in bone metabolism. While needed in smaller quantities, these minerals are indispensable for optimal bone health. Nuts, seeds, whole grains, and seafood are valuable sources of these trace minerals.

Understanding the synergy among these nutrients is key to crafting a diet that promotes bone health throughout your life. It's not just about individual nutrients but how they harmonize within your body to create a robust skeletal structure. Think of it as a symphony, where each instrument has a unique role, yet together they create a harmonious melody.

Incorporating a variety of foods rich in these nutrients ensures that you're not only nourishing your bones but also reaping the benefits of a well-rounded and balanced diet. Remember, it's not just about consuming these nutrients in isolation but embracing a holistic approach to nutrition that fuels not just your bones but your entire being.

As you embark on this journey of understanding the intricacies of bone-nourishing nutrients, consider this chapter as your guidebook. Armed with knowledge, you have the power to make informed choices that will not only fortify your bones but also enhance your overall well-being. So, let's celebrate the marvel that is your body and provide it with the nourishment it deserves. After all, strong bones are not just a testament to your physical strength but also to the care and attention you invest in yourself. Cheers to a future where your bones stand tall, supporting you in all your endeavors, and to a life lived with vitality and vigor!

Bone-Quality Feasts

The following are three example menus created by dietitians that give the suggested measure of day to day calcium.

The menus underline entire grains, vegetables, leafy foods and fatty dairy items. This assortment gives ample measures of calcium and different supplements.

Every day's menu depends on a careful nutritional plan of 2,000 calories, without any than 30% of the calories coming from fat. (Remember that you might require more calories or less.) Sodium is likewise restricted to 2,300 mg daily or less.

Menu 1
Breakfast

1 cup entire wheat chips grain, finished off with a peach

1 cup skim milk

2 cuts entire grain toast

2 teaspoons honey

1 tablespoon almond spread (no salt added)

Lunch

Turkey sandwich a la Mediterranean: 1 ounce turkey, 1 ounce part-skim

mozzarella cheddar, ½ cut tomato and 1 tablespoon pesto sauce on 2

cuts entire wheat bread

1 new apple

1 cup new vegetables: crude child carrots, celery sticks and broccoli florets

¼ cup without fat curds (plunge)

8 ounces cranberry juice (unsweetened)

Supper

4 ounces barbecued salmon steak

½ cup (3 little) broiled new potatoes

Spinach with feta cheddar and almonds (see recipe here)

1 entire wheat roll with margarine

1 cup skim milk

Nibble (whenever)

3 cups air-popped popcorn

Menu 1 healthful examination

Calories: 1,800

Protein, in grams (g): 99

Sugars (g): 276

Fat (g): 43

Soaked fat (g): 10

Sodium (mg): 2,175

Calcium (mg): 1,140

Menu 2

Breakfast

Omelet: 1 egg, 2 egg whites, 1 ½ ounces low-fat cheddar, ¼ cup cleaved onion and 1 ¼ cup hacked tomato; cooked in 1 teaspoon corn oil

1 little cornmeal biscuit

2 teaspoons natural product spread

6 ounces calcium-invigorated squeezed orange

Decaffeinated espresso with low-fat milk

Lunch

Veggie lover stew with tofu (see recipe here)

6 wheat saltines

1 cup slashed cauliflower and cucumber

¾ cup blueberries

1 cup vanilla sans fat yogurt

Home grown tea or other sans calorie refreshment

Supper

Barbecued chicken and vegetable kebabs: Marinate 3 ounces chicken in

pineapple juice. Stick and barbecue chicken pieces, chime peppers, cherry tomatoes and ½ cup pineapple lumps.

2/3 cup earthy colored rice, threw with parsley

2 cups spring greens with ½ cup orange portions and light vinaigrette

Water or other without calorie refreshment

Nibble (whenever)

2 ounces (½ cup) unsalted pretzel turns

½ cup plain Greek yogurt with dill (plunge)

Menu 2 healthful investigation

Calories: 1,900

Protein (g): 109

Sugars (g): 271

Fat (g): 47

Soaked fat (g): 14

Sodium (mg): 2,275

Calcium (mg): 1,422

Menu 3 (vegetarian)

Breakfast

1 cup calcium-braced soy milk

5 ounces vanilla soy yogurt with 2 tablespoons ground flaxseed and 1 cup blueberries

1 banana

Lunch

Vegetable, lentil and chickpea stew

1 entire wheat pita with ½ cup hummus

1 cup cut red chime pepper

Water or other without calorie refreshment

Supper

Tofu with bok choy

1 cup cooked quinoa

¼ cup sunflower seeds (dry-cooked, salted)

1 cup strawberries

1 cup calcium-sustained soy milk

Nibble (whenever)

1 apple with 1 tablespoon almond margarine (no salt added)

Menu 3 wholesome examination

Calories: 2,100

Protein (g): 87

Starches (g): 300

Fat (g): 74

Soaked fat (g): 9

Sodium (mg): 1,900

Calcium (mg): 1,500

Expanding Your Calcium Admission

Since it has become so obvious which food sources are high in calcium, work on tracking down ways of making these food sources part of your everyday eating regimen. Attempt to eat something like one serving of a calcium-rich food at every dinner. Three servings daily can give as much as 900 mg of calcium toward your day to day objective of 1,000 to 1,200 mg.

Think about the accompanying tips:

- Add 1 ounce — a cut or two slender cuts — of Swiss cheddar to your sandwich for an extra 200 mg of calcium.
- Get ready moment oats with low-fat milk rather than water — ½ cup of low-fat milk added to a parcel of oats gives around 150 mg of calcium. Braced moment oats give another 100 mg.
- Think soy. Numerous soy food sources are high in calcium. These incorporate edamame (new soybeans), normally found with other frozen vegetables. One cup has around 100 mg of calcium. Firm tofu can be utilized instead of meat, poultry or fish in a sautéed food, with around 250 mg or a greater amount of

calcium per ½ cup. Or then again nibble on soy nuts (dried soybeans).

- 33% cup has around 45 mg of calcium.
- Rather than sharp cream, which has little calcium and loads of fat, utilize sans fat plain or Greek yogurt as a plunge for vegetables and natural products. One cup of plain yogurt commonly has somewhere around 400 mg of calcium.
- Like Southern-style food varieties? One cup of every one of the accompanying has around 100 to 250 mg of calcium: cooked greens (turnip, collard, kale, beet or spinach), okra, dark peered toward peas and white beans.
- While making a smoothie, substitute ½ cup of low-fat milk, sustained non dairy milk or yogurt for water. Utilizing ½ cup of calcium-strengthened squeezed orange rather than plain squeeze

additionally will support the calcium content.

- You may likewise blend in a tablespoon of malt powder (50 mg of calcium) or dim molasses (41 mg of calcium).
- Utilize low-fat milk instead of water in soups. A 2-cup part of soup might give around 300 mg of calcium.
- Connoisseur treatment can add calcium. Serve eggs or fish on a 1-cup bed of cooked spinach for around 250 mg of calcium. Or on the other hand add 65 mg of calcium when you embellish vegetables or fish with 3 tablespoons of fragmented almonds.
- While cooking, recollect not to add milk to bubbling fixings or a burning hot skillet since milk singes without any problem. All things being equal, add hot fixings progressively to the milk, and afterward bring the entire blend up to temperature.

- Most recipes containing milk can likewise be cooked without singing in the microwave or in a twofold evaporator. While utilizing fixings that are high in corrosive, forestall turning sour by adding them to the milk step by step instead of the other way around.

Calcium Enhancements

In the event that you're not getting sufficient calcium in your eating routine, you might have to take a calcium supplement. An enhancement is frequently prescribed for postmenopausal ladies to assist with lessening the pace of bone misfortune.

Food sources to Stay away from

As well as realizing what sorts of food varieties and food fixings are great for your bones, specialists are likewise finding food fixings that can hurt your bones. There are a few food sources and refreshments you will need to keep away from or consume just sparingly.

Limit sugar, salt and phosphate added substances

Food varieties containing sugars that are added during handling for the most part give a ton of calories, added substances and additives yet couple of nutrients, minerals and different supplements. Consequently, dietary rules frequently suggest that you limit handled food sources and refreshments.

In the US, the No. 1 wellspring of added sugar in the eating routine is sugar-improved drinks. Carbonated sodas are among the most consumed drinks however regularly give almost no sustenance past sugar. Likewise, they might replace different beverages that could give calcium or protein to your eating routine. Also, improved tea and espresso beverages can add overabundance calories, possibly influencing your weight.

The Sustenance Realities name on most bundled food sources and drinks presently incorporates added sugars. Search for this number to figure out the amount of the all out sugar is normally happening, like lactose in milk, versus added sugars contributing void calories.

Most Americans likewise consume a lot of salt. The suggested everyday sum is 2,300 mg, which is identical to around 1 teaspoon of salt. The greater part of this salt is tracked down in handled food sources. Concentrates on show that elevated degrees of sodium are related with hypertension. Furthermore, an excess of salt expands how much calcium you discharge from your body when you pee.

Phosphorus, as phosphates, is utilized as an added substance in many handled food sources, for example, wieners, chicken strips, chips, handled cheeses and spreads, moment flavors, sauces, fillings and puddings, frozen items that are breaded, and cola drinks. An excessive amount of phosphorus in your eating regimen can impede how much calcium is assimilated through your small digestive system. To restrict your admission of sugar, salt and phosphate added substances, check the marks on handled food sources you purchase at the supermarket. While getting ready feasts, use spices, flavors and organic products to enhance food.

Limit liquor and caffeine

Liquor supplies calories yet a couple of supplements. It tends to be unsafe for some reasons when drunk in abundance, and certain individuals shouldn't drink by any stretch of the imagination.

Having more than one to two cocktails daily can add to bone misfortune and diminish your body's capacity to ingest calcium. Assuming you decide to drink, do it with some restraint.

Drinking liquor with feasts additionally eases back its assimilation.

Caffeine can marginally expand loss of calcium during pee, yet a significant part of the possibly harmful impact is expected to jazzed refreshments time and again being filled in for better beverages, like milk. Moderate caffeine utilization — around 2 to 3 cups of espresso daily — won't hurt you as long as your eating routine contains sufficient calcium. You can assist with balancing calcium misfortune to espresso drinking by adding a tablespoon or two of milk to each cup.

Recipes

Spinach with feta cheddar and almonds

Serves 6 (liberal ½-cup segments)

¼ cup fragmented almonds

1 teaspoon extra-virgin olive oil

1 enormous garlic clove, slashed

4 scallions (green nursery onions with tops), hacked

1 ½ pounds spinach, stems eliminated and very much washed in a few changes
of cold water
A limited quantity of water
Newly ground dark pepper
4 ounces disintegrated, diminished fat feta cheddar, at room temperature
Lemon wedges

Toast fragmented almonds in a sauté container over medium intensity until gently seared and fragrant. Set to the side to cool. In a similar skillet, heat oil, add garlic and scallions, and cook delicately for 15 to 20 seconds, being cautious not
to allow the garlic to brown. Add spinach and a touch of water. Cover and cook for around 1 moment. The spinach will wither quickly. Eliminate from intensity and top with dark pepper, feta cheddar disintegrates and toasted almonds. Embellish with lemon wedges and serve right away.

Supplement content per serving:

Calories: 140

Fat (g): 9

Immersed fat (g): 2

Cholesterol (mg): 15

Sodium (mg): 300

Calcium (mg): 190

Vegan stew with tofu

Serves 4

1 tablespoon olive oil

1 little yellow onion, slashed (roughly 1/2 cup)

12 ounces extra-firm tofu, cut into little pieces

2 jars (14 ounces each) diced tomatoes with no salt added

1 can (14 ounces) kidney beans with no salt added, washed and depleted

1 can (14 ounces) dark beans with no salt added, flushed and depleted

3 tablespoons stew powder

1 tablespoon oregano

1 tablespoon slashed new cilantro (new coriander)

In a soup pot, heat the olive oil over medium intensity. Add the onion and sauté until delicate and clear, around 6 minutes. Add the tofu, tomatoes, beans, stew powder and oregano. Heat to the point of boiling. Lessen intensity and stew for somewhere around 30 minutes. Eliminate from the intensity and mix in cilantro. Spoon into individual dishes and serve right away.

Supplement content per serving:
Calories: 288
Protein (g): 20
Sugars (g): 45
Fat (g): 5
Soaked fat (g): 0.7
Sodium (mg): 326
Calcium (mg): 195

Vegetable, lentil and chickpea stew
Serves 8

3 cups butternut squash (roughly 1 ½ to 2 pounds), stripped, cultivated also, cut into 1-inch 3D shapes

3 enormous carrots, stripped and cut into ½-inch pieces

2 huge onions, cleaved

3 garlic cloves, minced

4 cups low-sodium vegetable stock

1 cup red lentils

2 tablespoons no-additional salt tomato glue

2 tablespoons stripped and minced new ginger

2 teaspoons ground cumin

1 teaspoon turmeric

¼ teaspoon saffron

1 teaspoon newly ground pepper

¼ cup lemon juice

1 can (14 ounces) chickpeas (garbanzo beans), depleted and flushed

½ cup slashed simmered unsalted peanuts

½ cup slashed new cilantro

In a Dutch broiler, gradually sweat vegetables (squash, carrots, onions and garlic) over low to medium intensity until onions simply begin to brown. Work in vegetable stock and scrape up the seared pieces of vegetables on the lower part of the skillet. Add lentils, tomato glue and flavors. Cover and keep on cooking over medium-low intensity until lentils and squash are delicate (around 1 to 1 ½ hours). Mix sporadically. (Or on the other hand at this step move fixings to a sluggish cooker and cook for 4 to 6 hours on low setting.) Mix in lemon juice and garbanzo beans. Serve warm and finish off with hacked peanuts and cilantro.

Supplement content per serving:

Calories: 291

Protein (g): 14

Carbs (g): 43

Fat (g): 9

Immersed fat (g): 1.2

Sodium (mg): 182

Calcium (mg): 101

Tofu with bok choy

Serves 4

1 pound firm tofu, depleted

2 tablespoons hoisin sauce

2 tablespoons rice vinegar

1 tablespoon immovably stuffed earthy colored
sugar

1 tablespoon low-sodium soy sauce

1 teaspoon Dijon mustard

½ teaspoon stew garlic sauce

1 clove garlic, minced

4 heads child bok choy, split

1 teaspoon sesame oil

Heat the stove to 450 F. Cut the tofu longwise
into 4 cuts. Cut each cut into 2 triangles. Put
the tofu triangles on a plate and cover with
saran wrap. Top with a subsequent plate and a
significant burden and let represent 10 minutes
to deplete.

In a little bowl, whisk together the hoisin sauce, vinegar, earthy colored sugar, soy sauce, mustard, stew garlic sauce and garlic. Spread ⅓ of the blend in an elliptical baking dish. Channel the tofu, orchestrate the triangles in the dish and top with the excess hoisin blend. Prepare until warmed through, 10 to 15 minutes.

While the tofu is heating up, heat 1 inch water to the point of boiling in an enormous pot fitted with a liner container. Add the bok choy, cover and steam until delicate, 6 to 8 minutes. Move to a plate. Sprinkle with the sesame oil. Serve 2 bok choy parts and 2 tofu triangles on every individual plate.

Supplement content per serving:

Calories: 150

Protein (g): 13

Carbs (g): 13

Fat (g): 6

Soaked fat (g): 1.1

Sodium (mg): 438

Calcium (mg): 382

4.2: Exercise and Osteoporosis

In the quest for optimal bone health, exercise stands as a formidable ally, offering a multitude of benefits that extend far beyond the realm of physical strength. In this chapter, we will explore the intricacies of exercise and its profound impact on osteoporosis. We will delve into the two fundamental categories of exercises: weight-bearing and muscle-strengthening exercises, and balance and posture exercises. By understanding the science behind these exercises and incorporating them into your routine, you can fortify your bones, enhance your muscle strength, and improve your balance and posture, thereby reducing the risk of fractures and promoting overall well-being.

Weight-Bearing and Muscle-Strengthening Exercises

Weight-bearing exercises are activities that make you move against gravity while staying upright, forcing your bones and muscles to support your body's weight. These exercises are paramount for enhancing bone density and overall skeletal health.

1. Walking: The Simple Yet Powerful Exercise
Walking, a natural and accessible exercise, is a cornerstone of weight-bearing activities. Regular brisk walks stimulate bone formation, especially in the weight-bearing bones of the legs and spine. It is low-impact, making it suitable for individuals of various fitness levels.

2. Dancing: A Joyful Path to Stronger Bones
Dancing combines weight-bearing with rhythmic movements, making it an enjoyable way to improve bone density. Whether it's

ballroom, salsa, or even hip-hop, dancing engages multiple muscle groups and enhances balance, thereby reducing the risk of falls.

3. Hiking: Nature's Gym

Hiking not only offers the benefits of weight-bearing exercise but also immerses you in nature, reducing stress and promoting mental well-being. The uneven terrains challenge your balance and engage your muscles, making it an excellent choice for overall physical health.

4. Resistance Training: Building Muscles, Protecting Bones

Resistance exercises, such as weightlifting and resistance band workouts, target specific muscle groups, stimulating bone growth and enhancing muscle strength. By gradually increasing the resistance, you can build muscle mass, improve bone density, and boost metabolism.

5. Yoga: Harmony of Body and Mind

Yoga, with its focus on flexibility, balance, and strength, offers a holistic approach to bone health. Weight-bearing yoga poses like Tree Pose and Warrior Pose challenge your balance and engage your muscles. Additionally, yoga's stress-reducing benefits contribute to overall well-being.

Balance and Posture Exercises

1. Tai Chi: The Art of Balance

Tai Chi, an ancient Chinese martial art, emphasizes slow, flowing movements and deep breathing. Its graceful sequences improve balance, flexibility, and muscle strength. Regular practice not only reduces the risk of falls but also promotes a sense of calm and mindfulness.

2. Pilates: Core Strength and Alignment

Pilates focuses on strengthening the core muscles, enhancing posture, and promoting body awareness. By emphasizing proper alignment and controlled movements, Pilates exercises improve stability and reduce the strain on your bones and joints.

3. Balance Exercises: Stability in Motion
Simple balance exercises like standing on one leg, heel-to-toe walking, and balance board workouts enhance proprioception – your body's awareness of its position in space. These exercises challenge your stability, train your muscles to react swiftly, and significantly reduce the risk of falls, especially in older adults.

Incorporating Exercise into Your Routine: A Pathway to Stronger Bones and Better Balance

Now that you've explored the diverse world of weight-bearing, muscle-strengthening, balance, and posture exercises, it's crucial to integrate these activities seamlessly into your daily life. Here are practical tips to help you get started and maintain a consistent exercise routine:

1. Setting Realistic Goals: The Key to Long-Term Success

Begin with achievable goals tailored to your fitness level and gradually increase the intensity and duration of your workouts. Setting realistic goals ensures that you stay motivated and avoid burnout.

2. Finding Joy in Movement: Making Exercise a Pleasurable Experience

Discover activities that bring you joy – whether it's dancing, hiking, or practicing yoga in the comfort of your home. When exercise is enjoyable, it becomes a sustainable part of your lifestyle, rather than a chore.

3. Incorporating Variety: Spice Up Your Routine

Keep your workouts exciting by incorporating a variety of exercises. Alternate between walking, dancing, and resistance training to engage different muscle groups and prevent monotony.

4. Prioritizing Safety: Protecting Your Bones and Joints

Consult a healthcare professional or a fitness expert, especially if you have underlying health conditions or concerns. They can tailor exercise recommendations to your specific needs and ensure that you perform movements correctly, reducing the risk of injuries.

5. Consistency and Persistence: The Cornerstones of Progress

Building strong bones and improving balance require consistency and persistence. Stay committed to your exercise routine, even on days when motivation wanes. Remember, every step, every dance move, and every yoga pose contributes to your overall well-being.

In conclusion, the journey to stronger bones and better balance begins with a single step – a step toward understanding the transformative power of exercise. By embracing a diverse range of weight-bearing, muscle-strengthening, balance, and posture exercises, you empower yourself to lead a life of vitality and resilience. Your body, once nurtured through these exercises, becomes a fortress, capable of withstanding the tests of time.

So, lace up your walking shoes, unroll your yoga mat, and dance to the rhythm of your heartbeat. Embrace the joy of movement, the strength in your muscles, and the stability in your balance. With every exercise, you are not just building physical resilience; you are sculpting a life filled with vigor and grace.

Let your journey to stronger bones and better balance be not just a chapter in your life but a lifelong commitment – a commitment to yourself, to your well-being, and to a future where your bones are not just strong, but unbreakable; where your balance is not just stable, but unwavering. Here's to a life of strength, balance, and boundless possibilities.

4.3 Lifestyle Changes for Bone Health

In the pursuit of strong and resilient bones, making positive lifestyle changes is paramount. In this section, we will explore three crucial aspects: Smoking Cessation, Limiting Alcohol Intake, and Avoiding Falls. Each of these factors plays a significant role in determining the health of your bones, and understanding their impact is the first step towards a healthier, happier you.

Smoking Cessation

Smoking is detrimental to your overall health, and its negative effects extend to your bones. Research has shown that smokers are at a higher risk of developing osteoporosis compared to non-smokers. But why does smoking have such a detrimental impact on bone health?

When you smoke, the harmful chemicals in cigarettes interfere with the normal functioning of your body. Nicotine, in particular, disrupts the balance between bone formation and resorption. It hampers the ability of your bones to absorb calcium, a vital mineral for bone density. Moreover, smoking reduces the production of estrogen in both men and women, a hormone essential for maintaining bone strength.

The good news is that quitting smoking can lead to remarkable improvements in bone health. Within just a few months of quitting, your body starts to repair the damage. The increased blood flow enhances the delivery of essential nutrients to your bones, promoting healing and regeneration. As you embark on this journey to quit smoking, you are not just safeguarding your lungs but also giving your bones a chance to rebuild and regain their strength.

Limiting Alcohol Intake

While the occasional glass of wine might seem harmless, excessive alcohol consumption can wreak havoc on your bones. Alcohol interferes with the balance of calcium in your body. It impairs the liver's ability to activate vitamin D, which is crucial for calcium absorption. Additionally, alcohol affects the production of hormones, leading to decreased bone density.

Moderation is the key when it comes to alcohol consumption. For women, this means limiting intake to one drink per day, and for men, up to two drinks per day. By adhering to these guidelines, you can significantly reduce the negative impact of alcohol on your bones. Moreover, opting for bone-healthy beverages, such as milk fortified with vitamin D, can be a great alternative to excessive alcohol consumption. These choices not only promote bone health but also contribute to your overall well-being.

Avoiding Falls

Falls are a leading cause of fractures, especially among older adults. Preventing falls is essential for maintaining bone health and preventing osteoporotic fractures. As you age, your bones may become more fragile, making you susceptible to fractures even from minor falls. To safeguard yourself, it's crucial to take proactive measures to avoid falls and protect your bones.

Regular exercise is one of the most effective ways to enhance balance and coordination. Engaging in activities like tai chi, yoga, and strength training can improve your stability and reduce the risk of falling. These exercises not only strengthen your muscles but also enhance your proprioception, the body's ability to sense its position in space, reducing the likelihood of tripping or stumbling.

In addition to exercise, it's essential to create a fall-proof environment in your home. Simple modifications, such as installing handrails in the bathroom, securing loose rugs, and improving lighting, can make a significant difference. Regular vision check-ups are also crucial, as poor vision can increase the risk of falls.

Being mindful of your surroundings and wearing appropriate footwear are small yet impactful changes that can prevent falls. Opt for non-slip shoes with proper arch support, especially in wet or uneven terrain. Additionally, using assistive devices like canes or walkers, if necessary, provides extra stability and reduces the risk of accidents.

In conclusion, by quitting smoking, limiting alcohol intake, and taking proactive measures to avoid falls, you are not just protecting your bones; you are investing in your overall well-being and quality of life. These lifestyle changes might seem small, but their impact on your bone health is immense. Embrace these changes with determination and persistence, knowing that with each step, you are fortifying your bones and securing a future filled with strength and vitality. Your bones are the foundation upon which you build your life – nurture them, care for them, and they will support you in every endeavor, ensuring a future free from the shackles of osteoporosis.

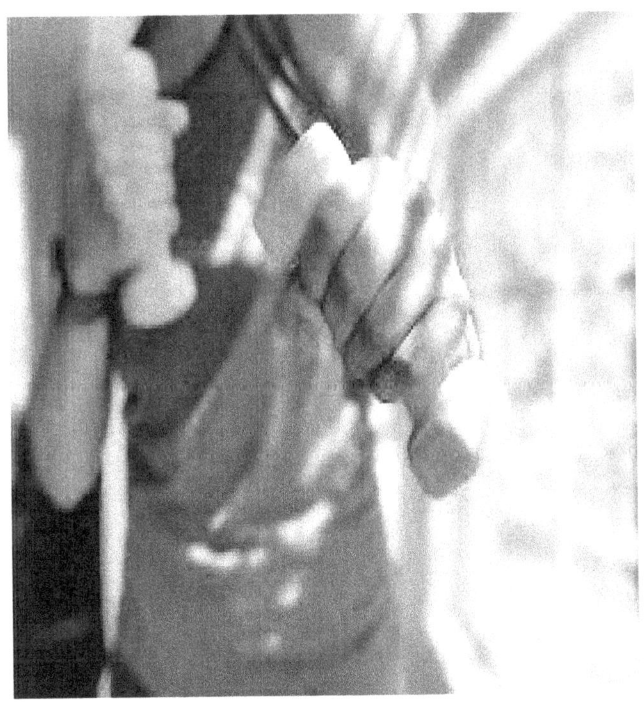

Chapter 5: Medical Treatments

In the realm of osteoporosis management, medical treatments play a pivotal role in strengthening bones and reducing the risk of fractures. This chapter delves into the various medications designed to combat osteoporosis, offering a comprehensive understanding of their mechanisms, benefits, and potential side effects. As you journey through this chapter, you'll gain valuable insights into the world of pharmaceutical interventions, empowering you to make informed decisions about your bone health.

5.1 Medications for Osteoporosis

When it comes to combating osteoporosis, medications are powerful allies. They work within your body, targeting specific aspects of bone metabolism to enhance bone density and reduce the risk of fractures. In this section, we'll explore three key categories of medications: Bisphosphonates, Hormone Replacement Therapy (HRT), and Other Prescription Drugs. Each category offers unique benefits and considerations, providing you with a range of options tailored to your specific needs.

Bisphosphonates

Bisphosphonates are a class of drugs that inhibit bone resorption, the process by which bones are broken down and their minerals released into the bloodstream. By slowing down this natural cycle, bisphosphonates help maintain and even increase bone density. Here are some commonly prescribed bisphosphonates and their unique characteristics:

- **Alendronate (Fosamax):** Alendronate is an oral bisphosphonate taken weekly or monthly. It helps prevent bone loss and reduces the risk of fractures, especially in the spine and hips. It's crucial to take this medication on an empty stomach, followed by a full glass of water, and remain upright for at least 30 minutes to prevent irritation of the esophagus.

- **Risedronate (Actonel):** Risedronate is another oral bisphosphonate available in various dosing schedules. It works similarly to alendronate, helping to strengthen bones and prevent fractures. It's essential to follow the specific instructions provided by your healthcare provider regarding when and how to take this medication.

- **Zoledronic Acid (Reclast):** Zoledronic acid is an intravenous bisphosphonate administered once a year. Unlike oral bisphosphonates, which require regular dosing, zoledronic acid provides the convenience of an annual infusion. It's particularly beneficial for individuals who may have difficulty with oral medications or prefer less frequent treatments.

Bisphosphonates: Benefits and Considerations

Bisphosphonates offer several advantages in the management of osteoporosis. By increasing bone density, they reduce the likelihood of fractures, especially in high-risk areas like the spine and hips. Additionally, these medications can alleviate bone pain and improve overall quality of life for individuals living with osteoporosis.

However, like all medications, bisphosphonates come with considerations and potential side effects. Common side effects include gastrointestinal issues, such as stomach upset or acid reflux, which can often be minimized by following specific administration guidelines. Some individuals may experience rare but serious side effects, such as osteonecrosis of the jaw or atypical femur fractures. Your healthcare provider will carefully assess your risk factors and help you weigh the benefits against potential risks when considering bisphosphonate therapy.

Hormone Replacement Therapy (HRT)

Hormone Replacement Therapy (HRT), also known as hormone therapy or menopausal hormone therapy, involves the use of estrogen and, in some cases, progestin to supplement declining hormone levels in postmenopausal women. Estrogen, a hormone that plays a vital role in bone health, helps regulate bone turnover and maintain bone density. Here's an overview of HRT and its implications for osteoporosis management:

- **Estrogen Therapy:** Estrogen therapy, available in various forms such as pills, patches, gels, or creams, provides estrogen supplementation to counteract the hormonal changes that occur during menopause. By stabilizing estrogen levels, this therapy helps preserve bone density and reduce the risk of fractures. It is most effective when initiated shortly after menopause, but its long-term use requires careful consideration of individual risks and benefits.

- **Estrogen and Progestin Therapy:** For women who have not undergone hysterectomy (removal of the uterus), combined estrogen and progestin therapy is often prescribed. Progestin is added to protect the uterine lining from the potential adverse effects of estrogen alone. While this combination can be effective in managing menopausal symptoms and preserving bone density, it also carries specific risks, such as an increased likelihood of blood clots and certain cancers. Therefore, individualized assessment and close monitoring are essential when considering this therapy.

HRT: Benefits and Considerations

Hormone Replacement Therapy offers multifaceted benefits beyond bone health. It can alleviate menopausal symptoms, such as hot flashes and vaginal dryness, enhancing overall quality of life for many women.

Moreover, estrogen supplementation has a positive impact on the cardiovascular system, reducing the risk of heart disease in some postmenopausal women.

However, the decision to undergo HRT involves careful evaluation of individual health factors and potential risks. Long-term use of HRT may be associated with an increased risk of breast cancer, stroke, and cardiovascular events. Additionally, estrogen-alone therapy can lead to endometrial cancer in women with an intact uterus. Therefore, it's crucial to discuss your medical history, family history, and overall health with your healthcare provider to determine the most suitable approach to hormone replacement therapy.

Other Prescription Drugs

In addition to bisphosphonates and hormone replacement therapy, there are several other prescription medications that can aid in managing osteoporosis and promoting bone health. These drugs work through diverse mechanisms, offering alternative options for individuals who may not be suitable candidates for or tolerant of traditional treatments. Let's explore some of these innovative medications:

- **Denosumab (Prolia, Xgeva):** Denosumab is a monoclonal antibody that inhibits bone resorption by targeting a specific protein involved in bone breakdown. It is administered as an injection under the skin every six months and is particularly effective in reducing the risk of fractures in postmenopausal women with osteoporosis and individuals undergoing treatment for certain cancers, such as breast or prostate cancer.

- **Raloxifene (Evista):** Raloxifene belongs to a class of drugs called selective estrogen receptor modulators (SERMs). It acts similarly to estrogen in some parts of the body, including bones, while acting as an estrogen antagonist in other tissues, such as the breast and uterus. Raloxifene helps maintain bone density and reduces the risk of vertebral fractures. It is also known for its ability to lower the risk of invasive breast cancer in postmenopausal women with osteoporosis or at high risk of breast cancer.

- **Teriparatide (Forteo):** Teriparatide is a synthetic form of parathyroid hormone, a naturally occurring hormone that regulates calcium and phosphate metabolism. Unlike other osteoporosis medications that inhibit bone resorption, teriparatide stimulates bone formation. It is administered as a daily injection under the skin for up to 24 months and is indicated for individuals at high risk of fractures or those who have not responded well to other treatments.

- Calcitonin: Calcitonin is a hormone that helps regulate calcium and phosphate levels in the body. While its effectiveness in preventing fractures is modest compared to other osteoporosis medications, it can be considered in specific cases, particularly when other treatments are not suitable or well-tolerated. Calcitonin is available as a nasal spray or injection and may be used to manage pain associated with acute vertebral fractures.

Other Prescription Drugs: Benefits and Considerations

The array of other prescription medications provides diverse options for individuals with osteoporosis. Denosumab, with its unique mechanism, offers a reliable alternative, especially for those who struggle with oral medications or have specific medical conditions that limit their choices. Raloxifene, as a SERM, presents a balanced approach, benefiting bones while mitigating the risks associated with estrogen therapy. Teriparatide, with its bone-stimulating properties, holds promise for individuals with severe osteoporosis or those who have not responded well to other treatments. Calcitonin, although less potent, can still be a valuable addition, especially when pain relief is a primary concern.

However, like all medications, these options come with their considerations and potential side effects. Denosumab use may be associated with skin infections, low calcium levels, and jaw problems. Raloxifene may increase the risk of blood clots and hot flashes. Teriparatide may cause dizziness and leg cramps. Calcitonin, while generally well-tolerated, may lead to nasal irritation and nosebleeds. As always, your healthcare provider will carefully evaluate your individual needs and medical history to determine the most suitable prescription medication for you.

In the realm of osteoporosis management, knowledge is your most potent weapon. Armed with an understanding of the diverse array of medications available, you are better equipped to navigate the path toward stronger bones and a reduced risk of fractures. Remember, each individual is unique, and what works best for one person may not be the ideal choice for another. Therefore, open communication with your healthcare provider is paramount.

As you embark on your osteoporosis journey, armed with this newfound knowledge, you are not merely a passive recipient of medical advice; you are an active participant in your own health. With the guidance of your healthcare team, you can make informed decisions, tailored to your specific needs and preferences. Whether you opt for bisphosphonates, explore hormone replacement therapy, or consider alternative prescription drugs, your choices are significant steps toward a life unburdened by the fear of fractures.

By understanding the benefits and considerations of each medication, you have taken a vital step toward empowering yourself. Your commitment to your bone health is an investment in a future where strength, resilience, and independence are your constant companions. As you move forward, let this knowledge be your guiding light, illuminating the path toward a life lived to the fullest, where your bones remain steadfast pillars, supporting your every endeavor.

Remember, your journey toward optimal bone health is not a solitary one. Seek support from your healthcare provider, connect with others who share your experiences, and embrace a lifestyle that nurtures both your body and spirit. Together, with knowledge as your ally and determination as your driving force, you can embark on this transformative journey toward a future where osteoporosis is not a barrier, but a challenge you have overcome, emerging stronger and more resilient than ever before.

5.2: Surgical Interventions

Surgical interventions are often considered when osteoporosis leads to severe bone damage, fractures, and chronic pain that significantly impairs a person's quality of life. In this chapter, we will explore two important surgical procedures: Vertebroplasty and Kyphoplasty, and Joint Replacement Surgery. Each of these interventions comes with its own set of considerations, benefits, and potential risks. Understanding these procedures can empower you to make informed decisions about your bone health and overall well-being.

Vertebroplasty and Kyphoplasty

Vertebroplasty:

Vertebroplasty is a minimally invasive surgical procedure designed to treat vertebral compression fractures, which are common consequences of osteoporosis. During vertebroplasty, a special cement-like material is injected directly into the fractured vertebra, stabilizing the bone and providing pain relief. This procedure is typically performed under local anesthesia, and the recovery period is relatively short, allowing patients to resume their normal activities soon after the intervention.

The process begins with thorough imaging, usually X-rays or CT scans, to precisely locate the fractured vertebra. Once the location is identified, a small incision is made, and a hollow needle is inserted into the damaged area. The cement-like material is then injected, filling the spaces within the fractured bone. As the material hardens, it provides structural support to the vertebra, reducing pain and preventing further collapse.

Kyphoplasty:

Kyphoplasty is a variation of vertebroplasty with an additional step aimed at restoring the vertebral height. Similar to vertebroplasty, it involves the injection of a special cement-like substance into the fractured vertebra. However, before the cement is injected, a small balloon-like device is inserted and inflated within the collapsed vertebra. This balloon helps to gently lift and restore the height of the vertebra to a more normal position. Once the desired height is achieved, the balloon is deflated and removed, and the cement is injected to stabilize the bone.

Both vertebroplasty and kyphoplasty procedures are highly effective in relieving pain caused by vertebral compression fractures. By stabilizing the fractured vertebra, these interventions not only reduce pain but also restore spinal alignment, allowing for improved mobility and quality of life.

Joint Replacement Surgery

Joint replacement surgery, also known as arthroplasty, is a common procedure used to treat severe joint damage caused by osteoporosis, particularly in weight-bearing joints such as hips and knees. This surgery involves replacing damaged joint surfaces with artificial components, which can significantly alleviate pain, improve mobility, and enhance the overall quality of life for individuals suffering from osteoporosis-related joint degeneration.

Preparation for Joint Replacement Surgery:

Before undergoing joint replacement surgery, thorough medical evaluations are conducted to assess the patient's overall health and suitability for the procedure. These evaluations include blood tests, imaging studies, and consultations with various healthcare professionals, including orthopedic surgeons, anesthesiologists, and physical therapists. Patients are also educated about the surgery, post-operative care, and rehabilitation exercises to ensure a smooth recovery process.

The Surgical Procedure:

Joint replacement surgery is typically performed under general or regional anesthesia. During the procedure, the damaged joint surfaces are removed, and the bone ends are shaped to accommodate the artificial components. The artificial joint components, made of durable materials such as metal, plastic, or ceramic, are securely implanted into the prepared bone ends. These components mimic the natural joint's structure and function, allowing for smooth and pain-free movement.

Recovery and Rehabilitation:

Following joint replacement surgery, patients undergo a carefully planned rehabilitation program to regain strength, flexibility, and functionality. Physical therapy plays a crucial role in the recovery process, focusing on exercises that improve joint mobility, muscle strength, and overall stability. Rehabilitation specialists work closely with patients to tailor exercises to their specific needs and monitor progress throughout the recovery period.

Benefits of Joint Replacement Surgery:

Joint replacement surgery offers numerous benefits to individuals with osteoporosis-related joint damage. It significantly reduces pain and inflammation, allowing patients to perform daily activities with ease. Improved joint mobility and function enhance the overall quality of life, enabling individuals to engage in physical activities, exercise, and social interactions without the constraints of chronic joint pain.

Risks and Considerations:

While joint replacement surgery is generally safe and effective, it is not without risks. Complications such as infection, blood clots, implant dislocation, and nerve damage can occur, although these are relatively rare. It is essential for patients to discuss potential risks and complications with their healthcare providers and follow post-operative instructions diligently to minimize these risks.

In conclusion, surgical interventions such as vertebroplasty, kyphoplasty, and joint replacement surgery offer hope and relief to individuals struggling with the debilitating effects of osteoporosis. These procedures, performed by skilled healthcare professionals, have the power to transform lives, allowing individuals to regain independence, mobility, and freedom from chronic pain.

By understanding the intricacies of these surgical interventions, you are better equipped to make informed decisions about your bone health. Knowledge empowers you to engage in meaningful discussions with your healthcare providers, ask relevant questions, and actively participate in the decision-making process regarding your treatment options.

As you embark on this journey towards a pain-free future, remember that you are not alone. A supportive network of healthcare professionals, family, and friends stands ready to assist you every step of the way. By embracing the possibilities offered by surgical interventions and combining them with a proactive approach to overall bone health, you can look forward to a future filled with vitality, mobility, and the freedom to enjoy life to its fullest.

With this newfound knowledge, may you stride confidently towards a brighter, pain-free future, where your bones remain strong, your joints function seamlessly, and your spirit remains unbroken. Here's to embracing life with open arms and a body that supports every joyous moment.

Chapter 6: Osteoporosis in Special Populations

Osteoporosis, a condition characterized by weakened bones and an increased risk of fractures, affects individuals across various demographics. In this chapter, we will explore osteoporosis in special populations, focusing on women and the unique challenges they face in maintaining optimal bone health. From the significant hormonal changes during menopause to the demands of pregnancy and breastfeeding, women navigate a complex landscape of bone health considerations.

6.1 Osteoporosis in Women

Women, throughout their lives, experience distinct hormonal fluctuations that directly impact their bone health. Understanding these changes is crucial in the prevention and management of osteoporosis.

Menopause and Bone Health

Menopause, a natural biological process marking the end of a woman's reproductive years, typically occurs between the ages of 45 and 55. During this phase, the ovaries cease to produce estrogen, a hormone essential for maintaining bone density. Estrogen plays a pivotal role in regulating bone turnover, and its decline during menopause leads to accelerated bone loss.

As estrogen levels decrease, bone resorption (the process of breaking down bone tissue) exceeds bone formation, resulting in decreased bone mass and increased susceptibility to fractures. Women undergoing menopause are at a significantly higher risk of developing osteoporosis. Therefore, proactive measures become imperative.

Strategies for Managing Bone Health during Menopause:

1. Dietary Choices: A balanced diet rich in calcium and vitamin D is essential. Dairy products, leafy greens, and fortified foods are excellent sources of calcium, while exposure to sunlight aids in natural vitamin D synthesis.

2. Regular Exercise: Weight-bearing exercises, resistance training, and activities that enhance balance contribute to bone strength. Yoga and tai chi are particularly beneficial for improving balance and reducing the risk of falls.

3. Supplementation: Consultation with a healthcare provider regarding calcium and vitamin D supplements is advisable, especially if dietary intake is insufficient.

4. Hormone Replacement Therapy (HRT): In some cases, hormone replacement therapy may be recommended to mitigate the impact of declining estrogen levels. However, the decision to pursue HRT should be made after careful consideration and consultation with a healthcare professional, weighing the benefits against potential risks.

Pregnancy and Breastfeeding

Pregnancy and breastfeeding are remarkable life stages, during which a woman's body undergoes significant changes to support the growth and nourishment of a new life. However, these changes also influence maternal bone health.

Pregnancy:

During pregnancy, the developing fetus requires an abundant supply of calcium for proper bone formation. To meet this demand, the body mobilizes calcium from the mother's bones, potentially leading to decreased bone density. While this physiological process is natural, it underscores the importance of adequate calcium intake during pregnancy.

Strategies for Maintaining Bone Health during Pregnancy:

1. **Nutrition:** Consuming a well-balanced diet that includes calcium-rich foods is crucial. Dairy products, fortified cereals, nuts, and leafy greens are excellent sources of calcium.

2. **Prenatal Supplements:** Prenatal vitamins often contain calcium and vitamin D supplements to ensure both the mother and the developing baby receive essential nutrients.

3. Exercise: Low-impact exercises, such as prenatal yoga and swimming, can promote muscle strength and flexibility without putting excessive strain on joints.

Breastfeeding

Breastfeeding is a natural and beneficial way to nourish infants, providing essential nutrients and fostering a strong bond between mother and child. However, breastfeeding mothers may face challenges related to bone health, primarily due to the nutritional demands of lactation.

Lactation and Bone Health

During breastfeeding, the body continues to prioritize the baby's nutritional needs, including calcium. If the mother's dietary calcium intake is insufficient, her body may continue to withdraw calcium from her bones, potentially leading to bone density loss.

Strategies for Maintaining Bone Health during Breastfeeding:

1. **Calcium-Rich Diet:** Emphasize calcium-rich foods such as dairy products, fortified plant-based milk, tofu, almonds, and leafy greens in the diet.

2. **Supplementation:** If necessary, calcium supplements can be considered under the guidance of a healthcare provider to ensure adequate calcium intake without compromising the baby's health.

3. **Regular Exercise:** Engaging in gentle exercises can promote overall well-being and support joint health without interfering with breastfeeding routines.

In conclusion, women undergo remarkable physiological changes during menopause, pregnancy, and breastfeeding. Understanding these changes and taking proactive measures to support bone health are essential for long-term well-being. By embracing a balanced diet, regular exercise, and, when necessary, supplementation under professional guidance, women can navigate these life stages with confidence, ensuring not only their own bone health but also the health and vitality of future generations.

As you continue reading this chapter, delve deeper into the nuances of osteoporosis in women and gain valuable insights to empower yourself and the women around you. Knowledge is the key to proactive health management, and in the subsequent sections, we will explore osteoporosis in other special populations, providing a comprehensive understanding of this condition and guiding you toward a future of strong, resilient bones and vibrant health.

6.2: Osteoporosis in Men - Causes and Treatment Options

Osteoporosis, often perceived as a concern predominantly affecting women, is a condition that knows no gender boundaries. While it's true that women are more prone to osteoporosis, men are not immune to this silent invader of bone health. In this chapter, we will delve deep into the specific realm of osteoporosis in men, exploring its causes, risk factors, and unique challenges. More importantly, we will unravel the diverse array of treatment options available, empowering men to combat this condition and lead lives unencumbered by the fear of fragile bones.

Understanding Osteoporosis in Men

Traditionally, osteoporosis has been associated with postmenopausal women due to the rapid decline in estrogen levels, which plays a pivotal role in maintaining bone density. However, men, too, undergo age-related hormonal changes, specifically a gradual decrease in testosterone. This decline, coupled with other factors, can lead to bone loss, making men susceptible to osteoporosis.

Causes and Risk Factors

Several factors contribute to osteoporosis in men, with age being a primary catalyst. As men age, bone density naturally diminishes, rendering bones more susceptible to fractures. Apart from aging, there are several other causes and risk factors to consider:

1. **Hormonal Imbalance:** Testosterone deficiency, often associated with aging or certain medical conditions, can accelerate bone loss in men. Low levels of testosterone compromise bone density, making men vulnerable to osteoporosis.

2. **MGenetic Predisposition:** A family history of osteoporosis can significantly increase the risk for both men and women. Genetic factors play a substantial role in determining bone health, and individuals with a family history of fractures or osteoporosis should be particularly vigilant.

3. **Lifestyle Choices:** Unhealthy habits such as smoking and excessive alcohol consumption contribute to bone loss. These lifestyle choices interfere with the body's ability to absorb calcium, a vital mineral for bone health, leading to weakened bones over time.

4. Dietary Deficiencies: Inadequate intake of calcium and vitamin D can impair bone health. Men with poor dietary habits, especially those deficient in calcium-rich foods and vitamin D, are at a higher risk of developing osteoporosis.

5. Certain Medical Conditions: Conditions such as rheumatoid arthritis, gastrointestinal disorders, and hormonal disorders can interfere with bone metabolism, exacerbating the risk of osteoporosis in men.

Diagnosis and Assessment

Diagnosing osteoporosis in men involves a comprehensive assessment, often beginning with a thorough medical history and physical examination. Specialized bone density tests, such as Dual-Energy X-ray Absorptiometry (DEXA) scans, are utilized to measure bone mineral density and assess the risk of fractures.

These tests help healthcare providers identify the extent of bone loss and formulate tailored treatment plans.

Treatment Options

Addressing osteoporosis in men requires a multifaceted approach aimed at slowing down bone loss, strengthening bones, and preventing fractures. Fortunately, there are various treatment options available, each designed to enhance bone health and improve overall quality of life.

1. Lifestyle Modifications:

- **Healthy Diet:** Adopting a balanced diet rich in calcium and vitamin D is crucial for maintaining bone density. Incorporate dairy products, leafy greens, and fortified foods into your diet to ensure an adequate calcium intake. Vitamin D, obtained from sunlight and dietary sources, facilitates calcium absorption and supports bone health.

- **Regular Exercise:** Weight-bearing and muscle-strengthening exercises play a pivotal role in enhancing bone density. Engage in activities such as walking, jogging, weightlifting, or resistance training to promote bone strength and balance.

2. Medications:

- **Bisphosphonates:** These medications inhibit bone resorption, preserving bone density and reducing the risk of fractures. Alendronate and risedronate are commonly prescribed bisphosphonates that help strengthen bones in men with osteoporosis.

- **Hormone Replacement Therapy:** In some cases, hormone therapy might be considered to address testosterone deficiency. Hormone replacement therapy can help improve bone density and mitigate the effects of hormonal imbalances.

3. Calcium and Vitamin D Supplements:

- **Calcium Supplements:** Calcium supplements may be recommended to bridge dietary gaps and ensure adequate calcium intake. It's essential to consult a healthcare provider to determine the appropriate dosage, as excessive calcium supplementation can lead to adverse effects.

- **Vitamin D Supplements:** Vitamin D supplements are often prescribed, especially for individuals with limited sun exposure. Adequate vitamin D levels facilitate calcium absorption and contribute to overall bone health.

4. Fall Prevention Strategies:

- **Home Modifications:** Making modifications in the home environment can significantly reduce the risk of falls. Installing grab bars in bathrooms, improving lighting, and removing tripping hazards enhance safety at home.

- **Balance Exercises:** Engaging in balance exercises, such as tai chi or yoga, enhances stability and reduces the risk of falls, which can be particularly beneficial for older men with osteoporosis.

Empowering Men for a Stronger Future

In conclusion, osteoporosis in men is a manageable condition, provided it is detected early and managed effectively. By understanding the causes, recognizing risk factors, and embracing tailored treatment options, men can fortify their bones and embrace a future marked by strength and resilience.

Remember, knowledge is your most potent weapon against osteoporosis. Stay informed, engage with healthcare professionals, and take proactive steps toward bone health. With the right approach, osteoporosis can be not a roadblock but a mere bump in the journey of life, allowing men to continue their pursuits with vigor, confidence, and unyielding strength. Here's to a future where osteoporosis is not a threat but a conquered challenge, where men stand tall and unshakable, embodying the epitome of strength in every sense of the word.

6.3 Osteoporosis in Older Adults

As we age, our bodies undergo numerous changes, and one of the most significant concerns for older adults is osteoporosis.

Bones, which once seemed sturdy and unyielding, can become fragile, making seniors more susceptible to fractures and diminishing their quality of life. In this chapter, we will explore the unique aspects of osteoporosis in older adults, taking into account the geriatric considerations and offering comprehensive strategies for managing osteoporosis in this vulnerable population.

Understanding the Aging Skeleton

Aging affects bones in various ways. Bone density naturally decreases with age, a process accelerated in women after menopause and in men due to hormonal changes. Osteoporosis, characterized by low bone mass and structural deterioration of bone tissue, becomes a pressing concern in the elderly. Understanding these changes is the first step in addressing the issue effectively.

Bone Remodeling in Older Adults: Explore how the balance between bone formation and resorption shifts in older age, leading to reduced bone density and increased fragility.

Impact of Aging on Bone Structure: Delve into the changes in bone architecture, such as decreased trabecular connectivity and cortical thickness, which contribute to the vulnerability of bones in older adults.

Geriatric Considerations in Osteoporosis Management

Caring for elderly individuals with osteoporosis requires a specialized approach, considering their unique medical and lifestyle needs. This section provides insights into the specific considerations essential for managing osteoporosis in the elderly.

Comorbidities and Polypharmacy: Understand the challenges posed by the presence of multiple health conditions and the use of multiple medications, and how they can affect osteoporosis treatment choices and outcomes.

Nutritional Needs: Explore the role of nutrition, including adequate calcium and vitamin D intake, in maintaining bone health in older adults. Learn about dietary modifications and supplements tailored to their requirements.

Exercise and Physical Activity: Discover safe and effective exercise routines tailored to the elderly, focusing on improving balance, muscle strength, and flexibility to prevent falls and fractures.

Fall Prevention: Delve into fall prevention strategies, encompassing home modifications, vision and hearing assessments, and assistive devices, to reduce the risk of fractures in elderly individuals.

Pharmacological Interventions in the Elderly

Medications play a vital role in managing osteoporosis, but their use in older adults requires careful consideration due to age-related changes in metabolism and potential interactions with other drugs. This section provides an in-depth analysis of pharmacological interventions specifically tailored for the elderly population.

Bisphosphonates and Other Antiresorptive Agents: Explore the benefits and risks associated with bisphosphonates and newer antiresorptive medications, emphasizing the importance of proper dosing and monitoring.

Anabolic Agents: Learn about the use of anabolic agents, such as teriparatide, in promoting bone formation, and understand their suitability for elderly individuals, considering their unique physiological characteristics.

Hormone Replacement Therapy: Discuss the role of hormone replacement therapy in postmenopausal women and its potential benefits and risks in the context of the elderly population.

Holistic Approach to Osteoporosis Management in Older Adults

A holistic approach to osteoporosis management in older adults goes beyond medications and exercises. It involves addressing psychological, social, and environmental factors that influence their well-being. This section explores the importance of mental health, social support, and environmental modifications in the overall management of osteoporosis in the elderly.

Psychological Impact: Discuss the psychological effects of osteoporosis, including anxiety, depression, and decreased quality of life, and explore strategies for providing emotional support and mental health care to older adults.

Social Support Networks: Highlight the significance of social connections and community involvement in promoting mental and emotional well-being among elderly individuals with osteoporosis. Discuss the role of support groups and social activities in enhancing their quality of life.

Home Safety and Environmental Modifications: Provide practical tips for making homes safer for older adults, including proper lighting, non-slip flooring, and assistive devices, to minimize the risk of falls and fractures.

In conclusion, managing osteoporosis in older adults requires a multifaceted approach that acknowledges their unique needs and challenges. By understanding the intricacies of aging bones, tailoring interventions to individual circumstances, and adopting a holistic perspective that encompasses physical, mental, and social well-being, older adults can continue to lead fulfilling lives, free from the constraints of fragile bones.

This chapter has explored the complexities of osteoporosis in the elderly, offering a comprehensive guide to understanding geriatric considerations and implementing effective strategies for managing this condition. As you navigate the pages ahead, remember that knowledge is power, and with the right information and support, aging can be a journey marked by strength, resilience, and vitality. Here's to a future where older adults embrace life with confidence, knowing that their bones, though weathered by time, remain steadfast pillars supporting a life well-lived.

Chapter 7: Living with Osteoporosis

Osteoporosis, with its silent infiltration of bones, often brings along an unwelcome companion: chronic pain. The persistent ache, the twinge with every movement, the discomfort that shadows your every day – coping with chronic pain becomes a crucial aspect of living with osteoporosis. In this chapter, we explore not just the pain management techniques that can provide relief, but also the essential psychological support that strengthens your resilience, empowering you to face each day with courage and determination.

7.1 Coping with Chronic Pain

Living with chronic pain requires a multifaceted approach that addresses not only the physical sensations but also the emotional and mental toll it takes. Osteoporosis-related pain can vary from dull and constant to sharp and acute, affecting different parts of the body, most commonly the back, hips, and wrists. Here, we delve into effective pain management techniques tailored to ease your discomfort and enhance your quality of life.

Pain Management Techniques

1. **Medications:** Your healthcare provider may prescribe pain relievers or anti-inflammatory medications to manage osteoporosis-related pain. These medications can help reduce inflammation and provide relief from discomfort.

2. **Physical Therapy:** A qualified physical therapist can design a customized exercise program to strengthen your muscles and

improve your posture, thereby reducing the strain on your bones. They may also use techniques like heat therapy or massage to alleviate muscle tension and pain.

3. Gentle Exercise: Engaging in low-impact exercises like swimming, tai chi, or yoga can improve flexibility, balance, and overall strength. These exercises not only relieve pain but also promote relaxation and a sense of well-being.

4. Assistive Devices: Using assistive devices such as braces, canes, or orthotic shoe inserts can provide support to affected joints and alleviate pain. These devices distribute pressure evenly, reducing strain on weakened bones.

5. Heat and Cold Therapy: Applying heat pads or cold packs to the affected areas can help relax muscles and reduce inflammation, providing temporary relief from pain. Alternating between heat and cold treatments can be particularly effective.

6. Acupuncture and Massage: Alternative therapies like acupuncture and therapeutic massage have shown promise in managing chronic pain. Acupuncture involves inserting thin needles into specific points on the body, stimulating nerve endings and promoting natural pain relief. Massage therapy helps relax muscles, improve blood circulation, and reduce pain perception.

7. Mind-Body Techniques: Practices such as mindfulness meditation, deep breathing exercises, and guided imagery can help you manage pain by enhancing your ability to cope with discomfort. These techniques promote relaxation and reduce stress, which in turn can alleviate pain perception.

8. Nutritional Support: A balanced diet rich in calcium, vitamin D, and other essential nutrients supports bone health and overall well-being. Proper nutrition can aid in the management of osteoporosis-related pain by ensuring your body has the necessary resources for healing and maintenance.

9. Sleep Hygiene: Quality sleep is essential for pain management and overall health. Establishing a consistent sleep schedule, creating a comfortable sleep environment, and practicing relaxation techniques before bedtime can improve the quality of your sleep, reducing pain-related disturbances.

Psychological Support

Managing chronic pain is not just about physical techniques; it also involves nurturing your mental and emotional well-being. Osteoporosis-related pain can lead to feelings of frustration, anxiety, and even depression. Addressing these emotional aspects is vital for holistic pain management.

1. Counseling and Therapy: Speaking with a mental health professional, such as a psychologist or counselor, can provide a safe space to express your emotions and develop coping strategies. Therapy sessions can help you navigate the challenges of chronic pain and build resilience.

2. Support Groups: Connecting with others who are experiencing similar challenges can be incredibly empowering. Joining a support group for individuals living with osteoporosis or chronic pain allows you to share your experiences, gain insights from others, and receive emotional support.

3. Cognitive Behavioral Therapy (CBT): CBT is a therapeutic approach that focuses on identifying and changing negative thought patterns and behaviors. It can be particularly beneficial for managing chronic pain by helping you develop healthier coping mechanisms and reducing pain-related distress.

4. Relaxation Techniques: Practicing relaxation techniques such as progressive muscle relaxation, guided imagery, or biofeedback can help reduce muscle tension and stress. Regular relaxation sessions promote a sense of calm, making it easier to cope with pain.

5. Expressive Arts Therapy: Engaging in creative activities like painting, writing, or music can serve as outlets for self-expression. Expressive arts therapy allows you to explore your emotions and experiences in a creative manner, offering a sense of control and empowerment.

6. Mindfulness and Meditation: Mindfulness practices involve being present in the moment without judgment. Mindful meditation can help you develop acceptance of your pain, reducing the emotional resistance that often exacerbates discomfort. Regular meditation sessions enhance emotional well-being and resilience.

Coping with chronic pain while living with osteoporosis is undoubtedly a challenge, but it is one that can be met with resilience, support, and the right strategies. By combining effective pain management techniques with psychological support, you can reclaim control over your life. Remember, you are not alone on this journey. Reach out to your healthcare providers, therapists, support groups, and loved ones. With the right support system and a proactive approach, you can navigate the complexities of chronic pain, emerging stronger and more resilient on the other side. Embrace each day with the knowledge that you have the tools to manage your pain and the strength to face the future with courage and optimism. Your journey toward pain-free living begins now.

7.2 Maintaining Independence

In the journey of life, maintaining independence is paramount. As we age or face health challenges like osteoporosis, the ability to live independently can be significantly impacted. However, with the right knowledge, tools, and support, it's possible to maintain your autonomy and continue living life on your terms. In this section, we'll explore two essential aspects of maintaining independence: assistive devices and home modifications, and community resources and support groups.

Assistive Devices and Home Modifications

1. Understanding Assistive Devices:

Assistive devices come in various forms, designed to enhance mobility, improve safety, and facilitate daily activities. From simple items like grab bars and walking canes to advanced technologies like stairlifts and mobility scooters, the market offers a plethora of options. We'll delve into the types of assistive devices available, their benefits, and how to choose the right ones based on individual needs.

2. Home Modifications for Safety and Accessibility:

Your home should be a haven of safety and comfort. Home modifications play a pivotal role in ensuring that your living space is conducive to your needs. We'll discuss practical modifications such as installing handrails, ramps, and non-slip flooring. Additionally, we'll explore the importance of proper lighting and how it can prevent accidents. Understanding these modifications not only promotes safety but also fosters a sense of confidence and independence within your own home.

3. Adaptive Technologies:

In our technologically advanced world, adaptive technologies have become invaluable tools for maintaining independence. We'll explore devices like voice-activated assistants, smart home systems, and wearable devices designed to monitor health parameters. These technologies not only enhance safety but also provide peace of mind, enabling individuals to live independently while staying connected to the outside world.

4. Financial Assistance and Insurance Coverage:

Acquiring assistive devices and making home modifications can be financially daunting. We'll provide insights into available financial assistance programs, grants, and insurance coverage options. Understanding these avenues can significantly ease the financial burden, making it feasible for individuals to invest in the necessary tools for maintaining independence.

Community Resources and Support Groups

1. Local Community Resources:

Your local community is a rich source of support. We'll explore community centers, senior services, and nonprofit organizations that offer various programs catering to the needs of older adults and individuals with health challenges. From fitness classes to transportation services, these resources can enhance your social interactions and overall well-being.

2. Support Groups:

Emotional support is invaluable, especially when facing health challenges like osteoporosis. Support groups provide a platform for individuals to share experiences, seek advice, and find solace in the company of others who understand their journey. We'll discuss the benefits of joining support groups, how to find local or online groups, and the positive impact they can have on mental and emotional health.

3. Counseling and Therapy Services:

Dealing with the physical and emotional aspects of osteoporosis can be overwhelming. Counseling and therapy services tailored to individuals facing health challenges can provide coping strategies, reduce anxiety, and enhance overall mental well-being. We'll explore different types of counseling services, how to access them, and the transformative effects they can have on one's quality of life.

4. Volunteering and Community Engagement:

Maintaining independence isn't just about receiving support; it's also about giving back to the community. Engaging in volunteer activities not only fosters a sense of purpose but also strengthens social connections. We'll discuss various volunteering opportunities and community engagement initiatives that allow individuals to contribute their skills and time, thereby enriching their lives and the lives of others.

In conclusion, maintaining independence is a multifaceted endeavor that encompasses physical, emotional, and social aspects. By embracing assistive devices, making home modifications, tapping into community resources, and engaging with support groups, individuals can lead fulfilling lives despite the challenges posed by osteoporosis. Remember, your journey toward independence is unique, and the support you need is readily available. By reaching out, staying informed, and staying engaged, you can continue to live life on your own terms, savoring each moment and celebrating your strength and resilience. Embrace the tools, the knowledge, and the community around you, and let your journey toward independence be a testament to your unwavering spirit and determination.

Conclusion

As we near the end of our journey through "Keep Your Bones Strong: Practical Approach to Osteoporosis, Improve Bone Strength and Reduce Your Risk of Fractures," you've gathered a wealth of knowledge about osteoporosis, its impact on your life, and the tools at your disposal to protect your bone health. The conclusion serves as a pivotal point in your understanding of this complex condition, combining the insights gained throughout this book and offering you a roadmap for taking control of your bone health. In this conclusion, we'll explore the practical steps you can take to fortify your bones, and we'll also peek into the future of osteoporosis research, providing a glimpse of what's on the horizon.

Taking Control of Your Bone Health

Over the course of this book, you've learned about the importance of maintaining strong and healthy bones, and how osteoporosis can threaten that foundation. Now, it's time to put that knowledge into action. Taking control of your bone health is a proactive journey that involves a combination of lifestyle changes, medical interventions, and a deep understanding of your own body.

1. Lifestyle Changes for Strong Bones: Your daily habits play a significant role in maintaining your bone health. We've discussed the importance of nutrition, exercise, and a bone-friendly lifestyle. In this section, we'll provide you with a detailed plan to incorporate these changes into your life.

a. Nutrition for Strong Bones: You'll receive comprehensive guidance on how to adapt your diet to ensure you're getting the essential nutrients your bones need, including calcium, vitamin D, and other important elements.

b. Exercise and Osteoporosis: Discover an exercise regimen tailored to your needs, with a focus on weight-bearing exercises, muscle strengthening, and balance and posture improvements.

c. Lifestyle Modifications: Learn how to make your home and surroundings safer, reducing the risk of falls and fractures. We'll also discuss the importance of quitting smoking and moderating alcohol consumption.

2. Understanding Medications and Treatments: In some cases, medical interventions may be necessary to manage osteoporosis. We'll delve deeper into the various medications available,

their benefits, and potential side effects. You'll gain insights into the decision-making process when it comes to treatment.

3. Regular Monitoring: Osteoporosis is not a one-time diagnosis but an ongoing journey. Regular check-ups and bone density tests are crucial for tracking your progress and adapting your bone health plan as needed.

4.Psychological and Emotional Support: Coping with a chronic condition like osteoporosis can be emotionally challenging. We'll provide strategies for managing pain, stress, and maintaining a positive mindset throughout your bone health journey.

5. Independence and Quality of Life: This section will empower you to continue leading an independent and fulfilling life, even with an osteoporosis diagnosis. You'll discover practical

tips for adapting your living environment and daily routines to support your well-being.

6. Community and Resources: No journey is meant to be walked alone. Explore the importance of support groups and community resources that can provide guidance, shared experiences, and emotional support.

By implementing the lessons from this book, you'll be well-equipped to take control of your bone health and significantly reduce your risk of fractures and complications related to osteoporosis. The power to strengthen your bones and enhance your quality of life lies in your hands.

The Future of Osteoporosis Research

As we conclude our exploration of osteoporosis, it's essential to peer into the future, where scientific advancements hold the promise of even greater understanding, prevention, and treatment of this condition. Osteoporosis research is a dynamic field, with ongoing studies that offer hope for individuals facing this challenge.

1. Emerging Treatments: Researchers are continually developing new treatments and therapies for osteoporosis. Some of these may offer more targeted and effective approaches to managing bone health.

2. Genetic Insights: Genetic research is shedding light on the role of genetics in osteoporosis. In the future, personalized medicine may become a reality, tailoring

treatment plans to an individual's genetic profile.

3. Advanced Diagnostic Tools: New diagnostic tools may provide more accurate and earlier detection of osteoporosis, allowing for proactive measures to be taken even before bone loss becomes severe.

4. Nutritional Breakthroughs: Ongoing studies explore the role of various nutrients and supplements in promoting bone health. Understanding these better may lead to more precise dietary recommendations.

5. Prevention and Education: Research in the area of prevention and patient education is advancing, with an emphasis on spreading awareness and teaching individuals how to reduce their risk of osteoporosis.

6. Bone Regeneration: Regenerative medicine offers the potential for growing and repairing bone tissue. This could be a game-changer for those with advanced osteoporosis.

While we can't predict the exact course of future discoveries, one thing is certain: the future of osteoporosis research is bright. As a reader of this book, you're positioned to stay informed about these breakthroughs, adapt your bone health strategies accordingly, and lead the way in taking control of your health.

In conclusion, "Keep Your Bones Strong: Practical Approach to Osteoporosis, Improve Bone Strength and Reduce Your Risk of Fractures" is more than a book; it's a resource, a guide, and a companion on your journey to better bone health. The journey doesn't end here; it's a lifelong commitment to taking care of your bones. With the knowledge, insights, and actionable advice you've gained from this book, you have the tools to lead a vibrant life, free from the shadow of osteoporosis.

Your bones, once silent and unnoticed, are now your allies. They will support you, just as the knowledge within these pages supports you. Let this conclusion be the beginning of a new chapter in your life, one in which your bones are strong, your future is bright, and your journey is filled with vitality and well-being.

Thank you for taking this journey with us, and may your path to strong and healthy bones be a rewarding and fulfilling one.